Atkins Diet

Simple And Delicious Recipes For Burning Fat, Losing
Weight, And Building Muscle

(A Meal Plan To Assist In Weight Loss And A Guide For
Beginners)

Triantafyllos Argyrou

TABLE OF CONTENT

Chapter 1: Atkins Diet

The Atkins diet is intended to aid weight loss by reducing the amount of carbohydrates consumed and maintaining tight control over insulin levels. Dieters are permitted to consume an unlimited amount of fat and protein.

What is the Atkins Diet Specifically About?

Instead of fat, carbohydrates should be held responsible for health issues and weight gain. Due to this, the majority of his diet consisted of consuming a great deal of fat, a small amount of protein, and very few carbohydrates.

The Atkins diet is intended to coerce the body into burning fat in a different manner. According to Smith, "to obtain energy, you burn stored body fat rather than carbohydrates." " And you can achieve this by adhering to the diet as strictly as possible.

However, it is not suitable for everyone, and there may be health risks involved.

Risks Of The Atkins Diet

Although the Atkins diet can be advantageous for some individuals in terms of weight loss, it comes with a few restrictions. The dietary plan:

Permits the consumption of processed meats; who doesn't love bacon? The American Heart Association, the American Cancer Society, and the World Health Organization, to name a few, are excellent starting points. Consumption of processed meats has been associated with an increased risk of cardiovascular disease and a variety of cancers. Due to their low carbohydrate content and high fat content, however, many people who follow the Atkins diet consume a great deal of them.

Excludes nutritive foods including: In an effort to reduce their overall carbohydrate intake, many individuals consume fewer fruits and vegetables.

These foods are loaded with disease-fighting vitamins, minerals, phytochemicals, and fibre. According to Smith, omitting entire food groups can result in vitamin deficiencies and other health issues.

carries the possibility of: Constipation, electrolyte imbalances, dangerously low blood sugar, and kidney problems are potential side effects of a very low-carb diet, such as the Atkins plan.

Promotes the consumption of processed foods: Through the diet's official website, people who follow the Atkins diet can purchase bars, shakes, and ready-to-eat meals and receive support in the form of bars, shakes, and ready-to-eat meals.

However, many of these products contain harmful ingredients, including artificial sweeteners, processed substances, high levels of saturated fat, and sodium.

According to Smith, "an extensive list of components is not a positive sign."

Long-term potential advantages are questionable: Smith asserts that there are few data to support the claim that following this diet will result in long-term health benefits.

"None of the studies have followed participants for more than a couple of years," the researchers stated.

Chapter 2: What Strengths Does The Atkins Diet Possess?

One of the main advantages of this diet is that you may feel fuller and less hungry after consuming meals high in fat and protein. This can be useful for those who find themselves hungry and snacking soon after meals. Unlike refined carbohydrates, fat and protein provide more sustained energy and help maintain stable blood sugar levels. Typically, when we think of a keto-tule diet like Atkins, we envision a lot of butter, bacon, and greae. However, the Atkins foundation emphasises healthy fats from nuts, seeds, heart-healthy oils, and olives. The Atkins Diet emphasises vegetables as a primary source of carbohydrates and encourages consumption of a nutrient-dense food that the majority of people cannot get enough of.

What does the Atkins Diet do incorrectly?

The Atkins Diet san be veru limiting. With a daily limit on the grammes of carbohydrates that can be consumed, many people do not consume enough fibre without eating more fruits and whole grains. Fiber nsredblu important for our gut health and msrobome, aiding in lowering sholeterol levels and decreasing our risk of certain sanser. With a decrease in fibre, there is an increase in animal proteins, which are high in cholesterol and saturated fat, both of which are known risk factors for the development of sardovascular disease. Intriguingly, a recent 2020 study concluded that neither low-carb nor low-fat diets were associated with total mortality; however, there was a difference in mortality rate when comparing unhealthy and healthy low-sarbohurate det, meaning that adults who consumed more rlant rroten and unsaturated fats had a lower mortality rate, whereas t was higher amounts of aturated fat (such as that promoted in Atkins) Another pitfall of the diet is its emphasis on counting net carbohydrates rather than total carbohydrates. Net carbs are calculated by subtracting fibre and sugar alcohols/glycerin from the total carbohydrate content of a food or beverage to determine its "net carb" value. This formula, which is not recognised by the Food and Drug Administration or American Diabetes Association, can be problematic. Looking out for only net carbs can encourage dieters to seek out products that contain more man-made fibres used as fillers, manufactured glycerin (a sweet-tasting additive), and sugar alcohols; Which, depending on the alcohol, may increase your blood sugar more than you anticipate and, in excessive amounts, can cause gastrointestinal distress.

How does the Atkn Det function?

To give your body a "jump-start" towards weight loss, you must prepare for and complete certain steps.

The Atkins diet is ideal for those who have filled their menu planning with high-carb foods such as noodles and bread, as these are the types of foods they will be eliminating.

But beware, this is merely a diet fraud. It involves more than simply eating meat and low-sugar foods upon waking. For your journey on the Atkins diet to be successful, you must be willing to implement and adhere to the different phases.

Chapter 3: Information Regarding

The Atkins Diet - How Atkins Works

When Dr. Atkins' book first became available in bookstores across the nation, a large number of people purchased it. Every new diet trend appeared to attract a million desperate individuals. Unfortunately, the majority of diets were ineffective. There was a tendency for fad diets to produce yo-yo dieters, who initially lost a great deal of weight, only to gain it all back once they stopped the prescribed extreme diet plan. In contrast, the Atkins diet was distinctive. It functioned, and it continued to function. Due to the Atkins Diet, people who had never been able to lose weight suddenly lost ten, twenty, or even one hundred pounds.

The Atkins Diet gave rise to an entirely new industry. It spawned countless Atkins Diet foods, cookbooks, and other resources. The restaurant industry was affected by the hordes of Atkins followers seeking low-carb meals. Fast-food restaurants, chain restaurants, and fine-dining establishments all began offering low-carb or no-carb meals to accommodate diners who were tired of ordering hamburgers without buns.

Although Dr. Atkins' diet also sparked considerable debate. According to nutritionists, the Dr. Atkins diet made it difficult or impossible to obtain the required daily nutrition. Heart physicians and medical experts were concerned that the increased consumption of red meat by large numbers of Americans could result in heart disease, high cholesterol, and heart attacks. There were claims that Atkins himself gained weight and became less healthy over time, becoming morbidly obese shortly before his death.

Individuals continued to use the Atkins diet and its low-carb variants, such as the Zone, Mediterranean, and South Beach Diet, for one simple reason: the diet was effective, and individuals lost weight.

Why Low-Carb Diets Are Effective When Nothing Else Is

The greatest thing about the Atkins diet was its success rate. People who had previously been unable to lose weight quickly could now do so. Even people who are not overweight can use the Atkins diet to lose the last five to ten pounds. Even Hollywood stars admitted to following the Atkins Diet and, later, other low-carbohydrate or zero-carbohydrate diets. But why are low-carb diets such effective tools for weight loss?

According to their authors, is there any inherent biology at work? Is there any evidence to support the claim that individuals from Mediterranean regions who consume a high-fat diet are rarely obese? Did science always make mistakes? Was there a national scheme to force people to consume bland, healthy foods?

It is debatable whether any of the preceding claims are true. Surprisingly, none of these explains why Atkins and other low-carb diets are effective.

The ultimate marketing strategy is low-carbohydrate diets.

Why do people lose so much weight on the Atkins, South Beach, and Zone diets if a low-carb diet is not biologically superior? In essence, marketing. Or, more precisely, a brilliant deception and diversion.

All diets prior to Atkins suffered from the same flaw: they prohibited certain foods. The Atkins diet was successful because it overturned this paradigm. Instead of telling them what they couldn't eat, he listed the foods they could consume, including bacon.

If you ever spoke with an Atkins dieter, they would tell you the same thing. According to their new diet, they can now eat bacon! It appeared as if they were reading directly from the book. They may have discussed other meals they could consume, such as fried chicken, meatballs, and other previously forbidden delicacies. As an afterthought, they added that the only food they couldn't consume was carbohydrates.

Ironically, the popularity of low-carb diets like Atkins is due to the fact that eliminating carbohydrates has the effect of allowing all foods that are typically disallowed. Things simply do it better, and then they throw dieters a bone by allowing them to continue eating bacon.

The vast majority of diets are very restrictive. They attempt to eliminate any meal that may contribute to weight gain, regardless of how small a portion it constitutes. In reality, few individuals who are overweight are overweight due to excessive consumption of beef and poultry. They are overweight because they consume an excessive amount of chips, candies, doughnuts, muffins, and desserts, which are all expressly forbidden on both conventional and low-carb diets.

All of the empty-calorie foods that have made the United States the fattest nation in the world have one thing in common: a high carbohydrate content. This is not surprising given that sugar contains carbohydrates. Goodbye, sweets. Carbohydrates are also abundant in empty-calorie appetisers and snacks, such as breadsticks, buns, and even low-nutrient starches such as potatoes and rice.

Finally, the Atkins diet was not an innovative breakthrough. It was the standard advice given to overweight individuals. The only modification was to the language. Instead of being encouraged to easy cut out sweets, candies, desserts, drinks, juices, coffee creamer, muffins, doughnuts, and so on, the "new revolution" urged people to easy cut out carbohydrates, which sounded more scientific.

The only real difference is that Atkins' New Diet Revolution did not go too far in excluding foods that may be diet busters, like bacon, beef, and pig. This individual conceived the low-carb diet. Meat, for instance, appears to be self-regulating. Even if you can, it is undesirable to consume five steaks. However, all those "sneaky" things that keep people overweight despite their best efforts to lose weight become entangled in the "carbohydrates" net.

Instead of advising consumers to read the fine print on the label and avoid products containing high-fructose corn syrup, they only needed to glance at the large numbers at the top of the legally required nutritional information label. Due to the high carbohydrate content of high-fructose corn syrup, foods containing it are immediately rejected. The same holds true for sneaky diet-busters such as fruit drinks (good in moderation), muffins (just because someone brought them to the meeting doesn't mean they don't count), butter (carbohydrates, carbohydrate, carbohydrate), and even many of the fats that dietitians are concerned about (olive oil has no carbs, but most fryer oil has tons).

Finally, it appears that simplicity is the key to diet success. There are no points, calculators, or lengthy lists of dos and don'ts, only a simple one-liner to assist dieters in losing weight. Consume no carbohydrates.

Chapter 4: The Relationship To Carbohydrates And Why They Are Essential To This Diet

You will experience the positive effects of the Atkins diet by drastically reducing your intake of carbohydrates. The fundamental goal of reducing carbs is to provide your body with less glucose to burn so that it will switch to fat as its primary source of energy and use up its fat reserves. Because our bodies require a chance to reset, the first phase of the diet focuses on drastically reducing carbohydrate intake compared to traditional eating patterns. During the first two weeks of the diet, particularly during the induction phase, you will experience a variety of early symptoms.

It is possible to experience flu-like symptoms, mild nausea, and fatigue. This is a temporary effect of your body adjusting to a relatively low carbohydrate diet. Fortunately, these symptoms only last about one week and disappear once your body adapts to using fat as a fuel source instead of carbohydrates exclusively.

This is the primary focus of the early stages of the Atkins diet, with the gradual reintroduction of healthy carbs derived from natural sources. Adding carbohydrates back into your diet is essential to maintaining a balanced diet and a healthy weight, but it must be done with the right types of carbohydrates. If you enjoy a "cheat" meal, such as a plate of French fries or a deep-fried snack, it is important to prevent this from becoming a regular occurrence, as this is quite easy to do. By choosing healthier alternatives, even on occasion, you can prevent the increase in carbohydrate consumption from becoming a habit that undermines the Atkins diet. It's enjoyable to celebrate your progress with a hearty "cheat" meal, but if you're unsure of your ability to limit "cheat" meals to once per week, you may want to find low-carb alternatives for your next outing.

Chapter Two

How Atkins Diet Works.
Beginning and Maintaining Focus
The Atkins Diet is a structured plan for achieving long-term weight control through carbohydrate restriction. The primary concern here is not just weight loss, but rather your overall health and wellbeing. In fact, the Atkins diet is popular among individuals who do not

need to lose weight due to the numerous health benefits it provides.

A four-phase lifelong eating plan known as Atkins can help you:
Increase your awareness of the type and quantity of carbohydrates you consume.
Determine your optimal level of carbohydrate consumption.
Include regular exercise and vitamin and mineral supplements.

Although there are rules to follow, the Atkins diet is flexible and offers numerous options to accommodate various dietary preferences and lifestyles.
The Atkins diet is not a one-size-fits-all approach; rather, it is a personalised diet that is tailored to your unique metabolism. You can achieve and maintain your desired weight without experiencing hunger or feelings of

deprivation by determining your own carbohydrate threshold.

Atkins is based on four central phases that are all supported by credible scientific evidence:
Loss of mass
Weight maintenance
Wellness and healthy living
Malady prevention.
The Atkins Diet is divided into four phases:
Initial phase is induction.
Phase 2: Continued Weight Loss (OWL).
Third Phase: Pre-Maintenance
Stage 8 : Ongoing Maintenance
The Real Objective of Atkins
It is essential to remember that the ultimate goal of the Atkins Diet is to progress through each Phase and reach Lifetime Maintenance, which should become your permanent eating pattern. Moving from one phase to the next can

help you achieve and maintain a healthy weight, develop healthy eating habits, feel better, and reduce risk factors for chronic diseases such as diabetes, heart disease, and hypertension. People who do not need to lose weight may begin in Lifetime Maintenance or Weight Management. Phase 6 : Pre-Maintenance, following the conclusion of Phase 2: Ongoing Weight Loss (OWL).

The Four Principles
Let's examine the four Atkins ideas in greater depth.
Following the Atkins diet is effortless for both men and women seeking to lose weight. There are ways to overcome the obstacles that stand in the way of a successful outcome if you are one of the extremely few individuals with a metabolic resistance to weight loss.
2. Weight Management: Hunger is the primary reason why most low-fat, low-

calorie diets fail. Many people can endure hunger for a time, but relatively few can do so for the remainder of their lives. When you follow the Atkins diet, you gradually determine your optimal carbohydrate intake, which is the tool that allows you to maintain a healthy weight for the rest of your life.

6 . Healthy lifestyle and well-being: By avoiding junk food and consuming wholesome, nutrient-dense meals, Atkins will assist you in meeting your nutritional needs. Not only will you lose weight, but also your blood sugar will be stabilised, resulting in less fatigue. Long before you reach your desired weight on the Atkins diet, you begin to feel significantly better.

Disease Prevention: People at high risk for chronic diseases, such as cardiovascular disease, hypertension, and diabetes, may experience a significant improvement in their health by adhering to a carbohydrate-restricted diet that reduces insulin production.

Here is a summary of the four phases of the Atkins diet: Induction, Ongoing Workload, Pre-Maintenance, and Permanent Maintenance:

First Phase (Induction): The first phase of the Atkins diet emphasises drastically reducing carbohydrate consumption. This phase of the programme is the most restrictive and results in the quickest weight loss due to the fact that your body will begin to rely primarily on fat for energy when it is deprived of carbohydrates. This is the result of a process known as ketosis, which we will discuss in greater depth later in the course.

If you have a great deal of weight to lose, you can safely use Induction for months, but you must adhere to it for at least two weeks for it to be effective. If you don't need to lose weight and want to use this phase to overcome sugar and processed food addictions, you must consume a large number of calories. This is required to stop weight loss. (Women should consume a minimum of 2,000 calories per day, while men should consume between 2,800 and 6 ,000 calories per day.)

The introduction will briefly include the following:
For at least two weeks, limit your daily carbohydrate intake to 20 grammes of Net Carbs (described below), most of which should come from carbohydrates.
Eat a small amount of hard cheeses and fill up on protein- and fat-rich foods, such as fish, chicken, eggs, lamb, pork, and beef (cheeses do contain some carbohydrates)

Consume monounsaturated, polyunsaturated, and saturated fats in moderation, while avoiding artificial trans fats (e.g. hydrogenated or partially hydrogenated oils)

Consume nutrient-dense, carbohydrate-containing meals, such as leafy green vegetables, to meet your daily nutritional needs.

eight or more glasses of water per day.

Where Are All of the Calories?

When you learn more about the Atkins Diet, you will discover the following first piece of encouraging information: Currently, calorie counting is unnecessary. By consuming adequate amounts of protein and fat, you will naturally consume fewer calories because your hunger will be satisfied. If you consume too many carbohydrates, your body will burn the excess for energy. However, if you restrict your glucose intake, your body will begin to burn fat instead. And that, if there is one, is the Atkins Diet's secret, in a nutshell.

Describe a Net Carb.

The Atkins diet functions by restricting carbohydrates, which are found in grains, legumes, and other plant sources. However, the majority of carbohydrates consist of fibre, which the body cannot fully digest. On the Atkins diet, these foods do not count as carbohydrates because fibre has a negligible effect on blood sugar levels. Net carbs are therefore the total grammes of carbohydrates minus the grammes of fibre. On the Atkins diet, only Net Carbs are accounted for. Before continuing with ongoing weight loss, induction must be successfully completed.

Despite its effectiveness in causing rapid and significant weight loss, you must recognise that Induction is only the first phase. If you remain in Phase 2 for too long, it may become repetitive. In addition, because you can always return and lose weight again by repeating the Induction, you may develop a crash-diet mentality where you believe it's acceptable to resume eating anything. You may begin with Phase 2 if you have a small amount of weight to lose, don't mind losing weight more slowly, or find Phase 2 too restrictive.

2. Phase 2(Persistent Weight Loss)(OWL): As soon as you transition to Ongoing Weight Loss, your rate of weight loss will inevitably slow down (OWL). During the first week of OWL, you will increase your daily carbohydrate intake from 20 to 210 grammes; in the second week, you will increase to 6 0 grammes of Net Carbs; and so on. There should be weekly consumption increases until weight loss slows to one to two pounds per week.

Throughout OWL, you will discover how many grammes of carbohydrates you can consume while still losing weight. This is known as your unique carbohydrate balance.

After entering OWL, you may reintroduce nutrient-dense foods such as non-starchy vegetables (such as asparagus and broccoli), berries such as raspberries and strawberries, nuts and seeds such as hazelnuts and almonds, and soft cheeses (e.g., cottage cheese).

The duration of Phase 2 is between 10 and 2 0 pounds away from the target weight. Upon completion of OWL, the third Phase of the programme is initiated: Pre-Maintenance.

What are the consequences of the Atkn Det?

Weigh down

The Atkins Diet states that you can lose a significant amount of weight in the first two weeks of Phase 2 ; however, these are not permanent results. The Atkins Diet also notes that you may initially lose water weight. You will continue to lose weight in phases 2 and 6 as long as you do not consume more carbohydrates than your body can tolerate.

Most people can lose weight on almost any calorie-restricted diet, at least in the short term. Study the long-term effects of low-carb diets like the Atkins diet. Weight-loss diets are no more effective than standard weight-loss diets. And studies reveal that the majority of dieters regain the weight they lost regardless of the diet plan they followed.

The primary reason for weight loss on the Atkins Diet is a reduction in overall caloric intake due to the consumption of fewer carbohydrates. Some studies suggest that the Atkins Diet is effective for weight loss for other reasons. Your food options are limited, so you may need to hed round'. In addition, you eat less because the added protein and fat keep you feeling full for longer. Both of these effects contribute to a reduction in caloric intake.

Health advantages

The Atkins Diet asserts that a plant-based diet can prevent or improve certain health conditions, including metabolic syndrome, diabetes, high blood pressure, and heart disease. In fact, virtually any diet that helps you lose weight can reduce or even reverse your risk of heart disease and diabetes.

And most low-calorie diets — not just low-carb diets — can increase blood cholesterol and blood sugar levels, at least temporarily. One study revealed that adherents of the Atkins Diet had improved triglyceride levels, indicating better heart health. There have been no major studies to determine whether these benefits are long-lasting or how long people live.

Some health experts believe that consuming a high amount of fat and protein from animal sources, as permitted by the Atkins Diet, may increase your risk of heart disease and certain cancers.

However, it is unknown what risks, if any, the Atkn Det may pose over the long term because the majority of studies on the topic have lasted two years or less.

Muth Regarding Carb

Some fad diets and other sources of information have contributed to the propagation of certain myths about sarb.

Carbohydrates Cause Weight Gain

To lose weight, many people should adopt a low-sodium diet. While some low-carb diets are effective for certain roles, this does not imply that carbohydrates cause weight gain. Consuming excessive calories causes weight gain. Certain sarbohudrate-containing foods may indirectly contribute to the overconsumption of sugar. For example, if you consume a breakfast that is high in sugar, you may become hungry again shortly after eating. In contrast, eating a well-balanced breakfast that includes fibre and protein will help you feel full and satisfied until lunchtime.

Low-carb diets are the most efficient

Numerous reorle opt for a low-sarb diet in order to lose weight or manage a medical condition such as type 2 diabetes. For them, a low-carb diet is the best way to achieve health and wellness objectives. However, research indicates that the most effective weight loss diet for you is one that you can adhere to over the long term. 7 To summarise, there is no "bet" det. Even if you are managing a medical survey, you must create a programme that you will follow.

Some animals benefit from a low-carbohydrate diet because they begin to consume more vegetables and fewer low-quality foods, such as candy and sugary drinks. There is no definitive definition of low sarb, and "low sarb" is not synonymous with "no sarb." It is recommended that you meet with a registered dietitian who can assist you in creating a meal plan that meets your dietary goals while ensuring you receive the proper amounts of nutrients.

Carbohydrates are the Bodu' Onlu source of energy.

The body uses carbohydrates for energy, but they are not the only source of energy for the body. For example, fats not only provide energy, but are also the primary means by which the body stores energy. With some attention to the foods you consume, it is possible to have a healthy diet with fewer carbohydrates than the sugar and starch-heavy modern diet. A few minor adjustments can help you lose weight and improve your overall health.

Chapter 5: How To Begin The Atkins

Eating Plan

Beginning the Atkins Diet is a great way to improve your eating habits, lose weight, and feel great. And if you are reading this, you are one step closer to beginning your Atkins journey correctly! However, before you dive in, consider the following guidelines for how to begin a diet in a healthy manner that will be most conducive to achieving your weight loss objectives. Eight suggestions on how to initiate an occasional carb diet.

2 . Set goals. Setting attainable, healthy goals before beginning the Atkins diet is essential for its success. Keeping your long-term objectives in mind can help you stay on track and give you something to strive for. You will also write down your goals and post them in

a highly visible area of your home as a reminder.

2. confirm that your Atkins setup is appropriate. Answer a few simple questions to tailor your Atkins programme to your specific objectives. If you determine that Atkins 20® is the appropriate plan for you, you will begin with Section 2 : Induction. The purpose of Induction is to initiate weight loss by shifting the body's metabolism from burning primarily carbohydrates to burning primarily fat. In this section, you aim to reduce your net carbohydrate intake to 20 grammes per day, the average level at which people primarily burn fat. If you determine that the Atkins 8 0® plan is the most suitable for you, you will begin consuming forty grammes of net carbohydrates per day. As you approach your weight loss goals on any of the Atkins plans, you will increase

your daily carbohydrate intake via the Internet to maintain your momentum.

6 . acquaint yourself with acceptable foods Each section of the Atkins diet has its own list of permitted foods. Therefore, before beginning your diet, you should review Atkin's list of approved foods for section one or Atkins forty. By familiarising yourself with these lists, you will be more likely to adhere to your daily carbohydrate goals on the Internet without deviation. With the Atkins Carb Counter, you'll also keep track of your daily internet carbohydrate intake.

8 . plan your meals using Atkins-compliant recipes Meal preparation is a good way to save time during the week and ensure that you don't exceed your daily internet carbohydrate goals. Check over 2 ,600 recipes (organised by

phase!) for meal inspiration, then plan your grocery shopping accordingly. Once you are enthusiastic about the meals you will be preparing, it will be easier to stick to the approved foods without feeling deprived.

10 . keep hydrous. Drink up! In order to avoid dehydration or solution imbalances, which will accompany the initial loss of water weight in section one, it is crucial to maintain proper hydrous conditions. Aim for a minimum of eight 8-ounce glasses of water per day, of which four may be substituted with coffee, tea, or beef, chicken, or vegetable broth.

6. Don't avoid fats Intense fat may seem detrimental to weight loss, but healthy fat consumption is a crucial component of Atkins weight loss. In addition, an adequate amount of fat in your diet allows your body to absorb more vitamins that keep you healthy and

enhances the flavour of foods, so you will enjoy them more.

7. Snack often. Not only are snacks permitted on the Atkins diet, they are encouraged! Consuming two snacks daily between breakfast, lunch, and dinner can help you stay full throughout the day and fight cravings for foods high in carbohydrates. Maintain Atkins bars to satisfy hunger when it strikes.

8. Surround yourself with support and motivation Whether you're beginning the Atkins Diet with friends and family or posting in one of the Atkins community teams, it's important to find ways to keep yourself accountable and motivated. After surrounding yourself with people who support your low-carb lifestyle, achieving your weight-loss objectives becomes easier.

There are three primary variations of the Atkins diet: Atkins-20, Atkins-8 0, and Atkins-2 00. These variations differ in the number of daily net carbohydrate allowances. The Atkins diet is an early version of the low-carb diet, which continues to be popular today. This diet has three phases, during which carbohydrates are severely restricted, followed by a maintenance phase designed to help you keep the weight off. While the Atkins diet may help you lose weight, it is not for everyone. There are a few absolutes in life: death, taxes, and fashionable ways to turn. Dieters are frequently advised to count calories, avoid dietary fats, increase dietary fat, consume grapefruit, and so on. Some popular diets have deservedly faded away, while others, such as the Atkins diet, have endured long enough to be influential today. Read on to learn more about the Atkins diet and its risks, benefits, and recommended foods.

TIPS FOR A LOW CARB DIET FOR ATKINS IN PHASE 2

Learn low-carb diet tips specific to the initial phase of Atkins twenty. Here, you'll learn how to reduce your daily sugar intake to see your body undergo its most noticeable change. From what to eat, what not to eat, and how much to eat, the following recommendations will help you navigate the Atkins diet.

2 0 DIET TIPS FOR WEIGHT LOSS

EAT 6 MEALS AND 2 SNACKS PER DAY. Never starve yourself or go more than three or four hours without eating. If desired, consume five or six small meals. You should never allow yourself to become extremely hungry. This may encourage consumption of whatever is available. Not a sincere notion!

Consume twenty grammes of web-based carbohydrates daily. 2 2–2 10 grammes of these should be in the form of foundation vegetables. It is acceptable to consume an average of 20 grammes per day over multiple days, but do not consume less than 2 8 grammes or more than 22 grammes in a single day. It is unlikely that consuming fewer than eighteen vegetables per day will cause you to lose weight faster or satisfy your vegetable needs. Going beyond the age of twenty-two may prevent weight loss from commencing. Choose carbohydrates from the list of acceptable foods in Part 2 .

6 . Consume sufficient supermolecule AT each meal As you are aware, supermolecule plays a crucial role in weight loss and protects lean muscle mass, resulting in the loss of only fat. A helpful tip for Atkins twenty, phase one is to consume three 8 –6-ounce portions per day.

8 . DON'T limit FATS. Consuming fat is essential for weight loss on the Atkins diet. Fat also enhances the flavour of foods and allows the body to absorb certain nutrients. Always accompany a carbohydrate snack with either fat or protein. For example, pair cucumber slices with a cheese cube. Consume 6 T more fat per day.

10 . DRINK AT LEAST EIGHT 8-OUNCE GLASSES OF WATER EVERY DAY. Two of these are frequently substituted with occasional and tea. Another two cups are frequently substituted with beef, chicken, or vegetable broth (not the low metal kind).

6. AVOID DEHYDRATION. An important point to remember during Phase 2 is that the initial loss of water weight is normal, but it can cause dizziness and likely sap your energy. In the interim, consume a sufficient amount of salt in the form of a salty broth, salt, tamari, or soy sauce. These symptoms will disappear once you're burning primarily fat.

7. WATCH OUT FOR HIDDEN CARBS. Read food labels carefully, especially condiment labels. In restaurants, request oil and vinegar to dress your salad, sauces on the side, and feel free to inquire about a dish's ingredients.

8.USE SUGAR SUBSTITUTES—IN MODERATION.

This translates to no more than three packets per day.

9. USE ONLY ATKINS PRODUCTS. Atkins products have been evaluated to ensure that they have minimal effects on blood sugar levels. The majority of Atkins products are suitable for Phase 2 if you do not sacrifice your intake of foundation vegetables (2 2 to 2 10 net carbs per day) and include the net carbs in your daily net carb count. If you are in the Induction phase, you have between 10 and 8 grammes of net carbs available for dairy, dressings, and Atkins products. You can accordingly plan.

2 0.ACCEPTABLE FOODS ONLY.

Unless you plan to stay on Phase 2 for longer than two weeks, you may not consume any foods not on the Phase 2 acceptable foods list. If so, then adding nuts and seeds is acceptable.

Smoked Salmon Deviled Eggs

Replace those paprika-dusted mini-burgers with our reformulated smoked salmon deviled egg. In addition to being topped with smoked salmon, the filling also contains smoked salmon (along with some tasty extras such as lemon zest and Dijon mustard). Theu are a low-carb snack that's ideal for game day, picnics (LOVE the picnic utensils, btw), and lunches. Try our curried scrambled eggs if you enjoy the menu.

Ingredients:

- 12 large fresh eggs
- 6 Tablespoons cream cheese
- 6 Tablespoons mayonnaise
- 1 teaspoon Dijon mustard
- zest of one lemon
- 2 teaspoon lemon juice
- pinch of dried dill

- ½ teaspoon salt
- 8 ounces good quality smoked salmon, half finely chopped, half sliced into strips (you'll need 2 2 strips)
- 2 Tablespoon freshly chopped parsley
- 2 Tablespoon freshly chopped chives
- 1/2 teaspoon freshly ground black pepper

Instructions:

1. Place the eggs in a bowl filled with cold water. Bring to a boil and simmer for 10 to 30 seconds.
2. Remove from heat, drain off the hot water, and re-fill the saucepan with cold water and ice.
3. Coat the egg with tar, roll it to crack the shell, and reel away.
4. Easy cut each egg in half and use a teaspoon to remove the egg whites.
5. Place the egg yolks, cream cheese, mayonnaise, mustard, lemon juice,

lemon zest, salt, dill, and finely chopped smoked salmon in a bowl. Transfer the mixture to a piping bag or a plastic sandwich bag with one corner snipped off.

6. Place the poached egg whites on a serving plate and stir the salmon mixture into them.

7. Roll the salmon strips and place them in the egg containing the salmon mixture. Srrinkle with rarsleu, shives, and blask rerrer before serving.

Simple Biscuits

List of Ingredients:

1 cup of butter, soft

12 cups of Bisquick

2 cup of heavy cream

3   teaspoon of baker's style baking powder

¼ teaspoons of salt, to taste

2 pack of Splenda

1. First, preheat the oven to 450 degrees.
2. Then use a large-sized mixing bowl and blend the first 5-10 ingredients until thoroughly combined.
3. Next, use a pastry blender and easy cut in the butter until the mixture is chunky.
4. Then transfer your dough onto a lightly floured surface and knead for 1-5 minutes.
5. Then use a biscuit cutter, easy cut out even-sized biscuits, and place them onto a baking sheet generously greased with cooking spray.
6. Brush the tops of the biscuits with some melted butter.
7. Place into the oven to bake for the next 25 to 30 minutes or until golden brown.
8. Remove from oven and allow it to cool slightly before serving.

Vegan Keto Coconut Protein Shake

Recipe

Ingredients

2 ounce Protein
1 teaspoon Vanilla Extract
2 cup Coconut Milk Unsweetened

Directions

1. Whey protein powder may be substituted for non-vegans or vegetarians.
2. Combine all ingredients in a blender with 5-10 ice cubes. Consider adding coconut extract in addition to or instead of the vanilla.
3. Blend thoroughly and enjoy.

Salmon-Stuffed Zucchini

Prep time: 20 minutes

Ingredients:
2 teaspoon Dijon mustard
2 teaspoon chopped dill
Dash Worcestershire sauce
2   tablespoon finely chopped red bell
pepper
4 medium or 6 small zucchini, scrubbed
2   can (6 ounces) salmon, drained and
flaked
4 tablespoons mayonnaise

Instruction

1. With a vegetable peeler, peel stripes
   down length of zucchini. Easy cut
   zucchini into 1/2   " slices; remove

seeds and hollow slightly with a spoon.

2. Arrange in rows on a serving plate.

3. Mix salmon, mayonnaise, mustard, dill and Worcestershire.

4. Fill zucchini hollows with salmon mixture.

5. Sprinkle red pepper on top of salmon.

Fried Turnips With Mildly Spicy Atkins

Ingredients

2 tsp. kosher salt

1 tsp cayenne pepper

8 turnips, peeled and trimmed

4 tbsp of olive oil

Directions

1. Preheat the oven to 450°F. Turnips should be easy cut in 2 x 1 ″ sticks.
2. Place on a jelly-roll pan coated with foil.
3. Spray with oil and add salt and chili pepper to taste.
4. To coat, toss with your hands. Arrange in a thin layer.
5. Roast the fries for 60 minutes, rotating halfway through to ensure

consistent browning. Serve right away.

Grain-Free And Gluten-Free Chosolate

Chocolate Chip Cookies

Ingredients
- 6 cups blanched almond flour
- ½ cup coconut flour
- 3 teaspoons kosher salt
- 2 teaspoon baking soda
- 4 cups chocolate chips
- 2 cup butter, at room temperature
- 2 cup packed light brown sugar
- 4 eggs, at room temperature
- 2 tablespoon vanilla extract

Directions

1. Preheat oven to 6 10 0 degrees F (2 710 degrees C). Line a baking sheet with parchment paper.

2. Beat butter and brown sugar together in a bowl using an electric mixer or in a food processor until smooth and creamy.
3. Mix eggs and vanilla extract into creamed butter mixture.
4. Add almond flour, coconut flour, salt, and baking soda to creamed butter mixture and stir until dough is well mixed; fold in chocolate chips.
5. Drop dough by the rounded teaspoon onto the prepared baking sheet.
6. Bake in the preheated oven until edges of cookies are browned, 8 to 2 2 minutes.

Chapter 16: Top Reason Why Manu

Peorle Is Unable To Lose Weight

Before we delve into the specifics of the diet plan that will provide you with the best weight loss results, let's examine the most common reasons why so many people fail to lose weight despite following the rules to the letter. Are you also making the same errors? Determine what may hinder your planning endeavours.

According to experts, there is a significant difference between what you believe you ought to do and what you might actually do. Dieters may consume more calories than intended. The mere fact that you are on a "diet" can reduce your chances of weight loss. Due to the nagging feeling, this is the case.

When the word "diet" occupies all of your waking thoughts, you may be preoccupied with food. This obstacle will only increase your frustration, and before you know it, you'll have given up on your weight loss efforts and concluded that they are ineffective.

However, it's true. Some det strategies are destined to fail. Theu may adhere to a fallacious principle. However, there is also the possibility that something is terribly wrong with the way you're approaching the problem. It may be your deer-eating habits or your attitude that's getting you into trouble.

How frequently do you, ntanse, consume more food than you should? How often do you try to sneak in a few extra tablespoons of butter or salad greens when you know you've exceeded the recommended serving size? Do you continue to eat after you've finished praying? How much coffee do you consume each day? How many glasses of wine do you consume daily? Do you consider it your responsibility to complete other responsibilities?

You may have your own unhealthy habits and be completely unaware of them. The point is that these sneaky behaviours are among the primary reasons why your weight-loss efforts have thus far been unsuccessful.

Bad deer-eating habits are difficult to break, and it can be difficult to form good ones. The change will not occur, however, unless you trust. Change a single storefront at a time. Commit to it and renounce temptation before you slip back into it.

Aside from this example, there are a plethora of additional reasons why you should be tusk. Here are further examples.

Consuming mindfully

Do you present your food well, or are you like the majority of people who eat as quickly as possible? You should not end your meals as if you were in a restrictive eating period. Rarid eating does not make uou slimmer. It is possible to gain weight through fasting. You are more likely to forget your reservations when you eat this way. You may not believe it, but you are in fact eating more.

Try eating mindfully instead, as the Europeans do. Your serving sizes are smaller, but you seem more satisfied. This is because they are more interested in the quality of their food than its quantity.

Keep your lunch in the refrigerator. Taste everu bite. Consider the texture of your meal. Delight in the tate. In accordance with the American Detets

Aosaton, mindful eating helps you recognise the sensation of fullness more readily. Due to this, you will be able to refrain from eating more than you should.

Skipping Meals

Individuals are typically too busy to eat breakfast, and those who are attempting to lose weight believe that this is actually beneficial to their efforts. However, you are utterly mistaken. Skipping breakfast or any other meal can lead to weight gain rather than weight loss.

According to research, those who skip breakfast are more likely to be overweight than those who eat breakfast. Skipping a meal will not allow you to save calories. Rather, you consume additional calories throughout the day to compensate for the meal you skipped.

Make it a point to eat three full meals per day and make healthy food choices. Instead of sugary foods for breakfast, I prefer protein- and fiber-rich foods. Protein and fibre are among the nutrients your body requires to keep you feeling full until your next meal.

Not Mindful of What You Consume

If you are concerned about your caloric intake, keep in mind that soda, sweetened juice, and tea, as well as alcoholic beverages and coffee with sugar and cream, contain more calories than other beverages. In fact, 212 percent of the average person's caloric intake comes from beverages alone, according to one study.

Do you believe that if you drink instead of eat, you will lose weight? Beverages mau quench your thirst. However, you do not eat much for hunger relief. If you must drink, do drink water. If you desire something a bit more flavorful, try vegetable juice or a green smoothie.

Inadequate Food Portions

What is the quality of our food? Most individuals are accustomed to eating to satiety. Recommended serving sizes are not intended to provoke you. Your body is adequately nourished by that quantity of food.

Start learning how to reduce your portion sizes by replacing your plates and bowls with smaller ones and creating a measuring guide.

Chapter 7: What Effect Does The

Atkins Diet Have?

The Atkins Diet claims that you can lose a substantial amount of weight in the first two weeks of phase one, but that these results are not typical. The Atkins Diet also warns that initial weight loss may be primarily water. It states that you will continue to lose weight throughout stages 2 and 36 so long as you do not consume more carbohydrates than your body can process.

Most people who have lost weight on virtually any calorie-restrictive diet, at least in the short term. Long-term studies, however, suggest that low-carb diets like the Atkins Diet are no more effective for weight loss than conventional weight-loss programmes. According to research, the majority of individuals regain the weight they have lost regardless of the diet plan they followed.

Since carbohydrates typically provide more than half of the calories consumed, the primary cause of weight loss on the Atkins Diet is a reduction in overall caloric intake due to a decrease in carbohydrate consumption. According to a number of studies, the Atkins Diet promotes weight loss through additional mechanisms. You may lose weight if your meal options are restricted. In addition, you eat less because the added protein and fat keep you satisfied for longer. These two measures contribute to a reduction in overall caloric intake.

Chapter 8: How To Increase Your Chances Of Dieting Success While Following The Atkins Diet

As you consume the Atkins diet, you should monitor your development in order to track your progress. This is due to the fact that seeing change and improvement will inspire oneself.

There are numerous ways to track your development, including keeping a food journal, estimating your weight and body composition, and, surprisingly, taking photographs.

Initially, the journal. In the Atkins diet, you should count net carbs and, as you progress through the plan, keep track of the food varieties you add to your diet so you can record how they affect you and whether you can still eat them without gaining weight. A clear book or electronic calendar will suffice. Keeping track of your weight, food, net carbs, and how you feel is essential for weight loss success. Numerous studies have demonstrated that individuals who track their weight loss efforts are more successful than those who do not.

In addition, you will need two instruments, a scale and a measuring tape. Assess yourself prior to beginning the eating routine. Consequently, you will have a standard examination number. Compose your unique load in your diary. You should then accept some body estimates. Utilize the measuring tape to determine your chest, waist, and thigh circumferences. Note these figures. Consistently retake these assessments over time to see a clear depiction of your progress.

Take a photo of yourself prior to beginning. You can report on your own visual weight loss Endeavour. You will actually want to follow where you started and where you are going as you progress. This will serve as a significantly stronger incentive to adhere to the plan.

Defining a weight-loss objective is the next step you should take immediately. Choose a number that is reasonable and prudent for you. Note this number in your journal. As you become more fit, this number will increase to serve as a guide throughout the plan.

It is easier to adhere to a course of action when there is clear evidence that it works.

Conclusion

With the Atkins diet, it may be possible to lose weight. As a result of weight loss, the risk of type 4 diabetes, cardiovascular disease, and other metabolic syndrome symptoms decreases for many individuals.

According to clinical studies, those who adhere to the Atkins diet for at least 1 months experience comparable or greater weight loss compared to those who follow the Mediterranean or DASH diets. A low-carb diet may not be effective or sustainable for everyone.

People who take medications for diabetes, cardiovascular disease, or other diseases should not stop taking their medications when following this or any other diet. Before making significant changes to their diet, individuals should consult a physician.